Anonymus

The medical profession and its morality

Anonymus

The medical profession and its morality

ISBN/EAN: 9783742832894

Manufactured in Europe, USA, Canada, Australia, Japa

Cover: Foto ©Lupo / pixelio.de

Manufactured and distributed by brebook publishing software
(www.brebook.com)

Anonymus

The medical profession and its morality

THE

MEDICAL PROFESSION

AND ITS

MORALITY.

.

[Reprinted with Corrections and Additions from

THE MODERN REVIEW, *April, 1881.*]

PROVIDENCE:

SNOW & FARNHAM.

1892.

PREFACE.

THE article, of which this pamphlet is an enlarged reprint, was answered in the next number of the same *Review*, July, 1881, by the late Dr. W. B. Carpenter, and by "Two of the Profession." A third article, which it was hoped would deal out justice in the controversy, was devoted by its writer merely to throwing oil on the waters.

In the present reprint, a few small errors noted by the former critics have been corrected. It has not been thought necessary to take much notice of their reckless, flat denials of many notorious, or easily proveable, facts, such as the general rowdyism of medical students, the history of the Vivisection Act of 1876, the prevalence of medical love-making in recent novels, &c., &c.

Reviewing the paper after the lapse of five years, the author feels afresh impressed by the urgent need of public attention to the charges made therein;—charges, it may be added, of which the heaviest are now corroborated by extracts from recent Addresses and articles by the leaders, and in the accredited organs of the Profession itself.

November, 1886.

THE MEDICAL PROFESSION
AND ITS MORALITY.

ONE profession amongst all those exercised in this
country has importantly shifted its position during
the past century. The Army, the Navy, the Church, and the
Bar stand much where they stood in the days of the Tudors;
but Edward IV.'s "Corporation of Barber-Surgeons" has
made a wonderful ascent from its pristine *status*, passing
up from Henry VIII.'s "Incorporated Society of Surgeons"
to the "College of Surgeons," as it exists in the reign of
Victoria.* A parallel elevation has taken place at the same
time in the other branch of the medical profession which
previously occupied (so far as its rank and file were concerned)
a very humble position, even while a few eminent men in
each generation rose to wealth and honour. At last the
ignoble squabbles of the surgeons with the physicians, and
of both with the apothecaries, are husLed, and the united
professors of the Healing Art have lifted themselves as a
body altogether to a higher plane than they ever before
occupied. By dint of cohesion and generalship they form
a compact phalanx, and have obviously suddenly arrived
at the consciousness of corporate power. The Medical
Council, already far ahead of Convocation, has become a

---

* The Incorporated Surgeons grew out of the Barber-Surgeons, and in its
turn became the origin of the College of Surgeons. In 1797, Lord Thurlow,
in opposing the Bill for the incorporation of the latter, was rude enough to
observe that "by a law still in force the barbers and the surgeons must each
use a pole," and that the pole of the surgeons must terminate in a gallipot
and a red rag. He would be a bolder Chancellor than Thurlow who, in
1886, would not tremble on the woolsack ere he reminded the surgeons of
our day of the pole and the gallipot.

little Parliament, destined soon to dictate to the larger
Senate of the kingdom, not only concerning its own interior
affairs, but also concerning everything which can by possibility be represented as affecting the interests of public
health.* As medical officers in parishes and unions, factory
and prison surgeons, public vaccinators, medical officers of
health, and very commonly as coroners, the doctors are daily
assuming authority which, at first, perhaps, legitimate and
beneficial, has a prevailing tendency to become meddling and
despotic. In the Army and Navy the surgeons, long unfairly
deconsidered, now haughtily claim equally unreasonable
precedence. Even the Government of the country appears
unequal to the task of contending with the profession since
Sir Richard Cross succumbed to the deputation which
invaded the Home Office many hundreds strong, and reduced
him to the humiliating concession of turning his own
Vivisection Bill from a measure to protect animals into
one to protect physiologists. The tone of bullying adopted
by the medical Press when the Government presumed at its
own discretion to appoint a Registrar-General who happened
not to be a doctor, was apparently intended to strike terror
into the hearts of any Ministry which should venture again
on such a step ; and the same may be said of repeated
efforts to insist on the penalties to be inflicted on the
heretic victims of these modern Inquisitors, namely the
parents who refuse to allow their children to be vaccinated.
In all newspaper correspondence, indeed, wherein medical
men express their views, a new tone of dominance, not to say
arrogance, is perceptible ; nor do many lay writers on the
press, or speakers in public meetings, venture to allude to the
profession without a sort of rhetorical genuflexion, such as
a Roman Catholic pays *en passant* in referring to the Pope

---

* A critic of this paper (*Modern Review*, July, 1881) scoffs at this remark,
and ranks the Council "the biggest sham in England—nothing but the
embodiment of a wind-bag."

or the saints. At the meeting of the Birmingham Branch
of the British Medical Association on the 29th June, 1883,
the President. Dr. Balthasar Foster, complained that "in
the House of Lords they (the doctors) had no vote where
the Church had its Bench of Bishops, and where the public
service of lawyers found their final recognition." But the
Birmingham Branch President was modest beside the
President of the Association, Dr. A. T. Waters, who con-
cluded his inaugural address at Liverpool, July 31st, by
saying (as reported next day in the *Standard*): "Amongst
the many changes which revolving years would bring, might
they not hope that .... there would come a fuller recognition of the claims of its members to some of the higher
honours of the State? The presence of medical men in the
House of Lords would *strengthen the powers of that House*
and beneficially influence legislation."

Literature, as usual, reflects in its waters the growth of
the aspiring tower on its banks, and represents the heroines
of at least half the novels of the last decade as passionately
adoring their doctors, to the cruel disparagement of all the
gallant soldiers and pious clergymen, who, in the earlier
years of the century, were understood to command the
affections of the romantic sex. As it will generally be
admitted, even by those who most highly esteem the
profession, that a lady's medical adviser is the last person
with whom it is natural or desirable that she should associate
the notion of love-making, this favourite modern legend of
Dr. Cupid and Miss Psyche speaks volumes for the space
now occupied by the professors of medicine in the popular
mind.

This universal uprising of the practitioners of the Healing
Art has naturally gone on *pari passu* with an increase among
the laity of care for bodily health and ease. It would seem
as if our ancestors scarcely realised how painful is sickness,
how precious is life—so enhanced is our dread of disease,

so desperately anxious are we to postpone the hour of
dissolution! As old Selden said, "To preach long, loud,
and damnation is the way to be cried up. We love a man
that damns us, and run after him to save us." "To preach
long, loud, and *sanitation* " is the modern doctor's version of
this apophthegm, and we do "cry them up," and run after them
to save us from " germs," and all other imps of the scientific
imagination. No one can foresee to what lengths our
poltroonery may go in this direction under the energetic
preachments of such Boanerges as Mr. Huxley and Dr.
Richardson. The thunders of the divines have long sunk to
a far-off roll of old formulæ, reverberated down the ages and
able to disturb us no more. But the claps of the sanitarians
are fresh and strong, and we tremble as we hear them ; for,
though we believe little concerning our souls, we have a
lively faith in our bodies, and generally follow the example
of the French lady whose epitaph records that she

Pour plus de securité
Fit son paradis dans ce monde.

In short, in every department of public and private life, the
doctors are acquiring power and influence, and coming to
the front. They are new pilots who have boarded our ship
and will shortly have a very large share of the handling of
the helm. It is a matter of deep importance to us to know
who and what manner of men they are and towards which
point of the moral compass they will guide us.*

First, who are the Doctors of Great Britain in 1886 ?
From what class of Society are they recruited ? Why do

* It may be suggested that another reason for the increased honour paid
to doctors by our generation is due to the fact that they have ceased to be
empirics, and become true men of science, and that they really are able to
cure us better than their predecessors. Such is, of course, the common
belief ; but it would seem that the faith of each generation of patients in its
own generation of doctors had been always as high as it could possibly be,
whether those doctors were the veriest quacks or the reverse. Each one has

they choose their profession? What is their education and general moral status?

I·, America and in several countries in Europe medical men often belong, by birth, to the "Upper Ten." It is not uncommon for French nobles in these latter days to be doctors, and we have lately heard of a German Prince adopting the profession. In Italy—ruled as it now is to a disastrous extent by "Professors" of all kinds—the doctors naturally take large share in the Government. In England, on the other hand (as is generally known, and as the Medical Directory proves), it has not been customary for men of the higher ranks to send their sons to King's College or Guy's instead of to Eton or Christchurch. The Hon. Dr. Herbert, Lord Carnarvon's brother, is mentioned so frequently in this relation that it would seem he must stand almost alone of men of his grade in the medical profession, while the Army and Navy and Clerical Lists swarm with the noblest names in the land. As a rule, it appears that the majority of British doctors are either the sons of men of the secondary professional classes or of tradesmen, and in some cases (especially in Scotland) of intelligent artizans. In Wales cases are not infrequent of doctors who themselves exercised humble trades, or were even domestic servants.

Much credit is due to medical men for the honourable ambi-

seen new remedies puffed by the faculty, and' old remedies falling into discredit; and we may say in our day as safely as Voltaire did in his time, that a doctor is a man who pours drugs of which he knows little into stomachs of which he knows less. If science, with all its boasting, and after its hecatombs of bloody sacrifices, had really made important advances in therapeutics, we should at least be able to point to some one or two unquestionable specific remedies for the most terrible scourges of mortality, such as cholera, or consumption, or cancer. Nothing of the kind, however, has been heard of; and it is even asserted, on respectable authority and with reference to registrar-generals' reports, that the mortality from the principal organic diseases is actually at a rate *far greater* in England to-day than it was thirty years ago. On this matter we do not pronounce an opinion.

tion wherewith they have stepped upward; but it is well to
bear in mind that they generally enter society (whenever they
attain its higher levels) by right only of their personal and
professional merits; and that they do not necessarily bring
with them quite the same set of ideas on all subjects as are
current among the young men educated in the great public
schools or older universities.   In no invidious sense, but as
a simple matter of fact, they should be understood to be a
parvenu profession, with the merits and the defects of the
class.   Thus they are more apt to hang together, and make
common cause against outsiders, than even the lawyers.
That there are hundreds of medical men in the truest sense
"gentlemen," judged either by the most conventional or
the loftiest standard, we all know from experience.   But
entry into the profession of medicine cannot be said (as
Rochefoucauld remarked long ago happened in the case of
the profession of arms) to make a man lose his vulgarity or
his coarseness, if he be originally coarse or vulgar-minded. *
    The motives which lead men to become physicians or
surgeons are not far to seek.   The average income of the
British doctor is said to be £50 a year higher than that of
the British parson, and less dependent on the chance of
patronage.   The pecuniary prizes within reach of a successful
surgeon or physician are enormous; and, though no peerage

---

* The lady who sits at dinner beside a new acquaintance—be he squire or
parson, barrister or soldier—rightly accepts any serious assurance he may
give her of facts under his own cognizance, knowing very well that the word
of an English gentleman is, as a rule, to be trusted, and that he has pretty
well learned at Harrow and Eton, Christchurch or Trinity, to regard a lie as
the forfeiture of his caste.   But when the stranger happens to be an eminent
Physician or Surgeon, it must be questioned whether she may equally take it
for granted that he will not tell fibs about many subjects (e.g., vivisection or
vaccination) on which they may discourse.   The speaker's manners may be quite
as polished as those of the peer or the guardsman, but he was neither born to
similar traditions nor educated in the same atmosphere; and it is to make a
silly mistake to forget the fact.   He may be a more truthful,—a more con-
scientiously truthful—man than any of the others, but, if so, it is by personal
merit alone.   There is no d *priori* presumption that truthfulness is ingrained
in his habits.

has yet been given to a doctor, the "Bloody Hand" of a Baronet holds out considerable attraction. Finally, beside such mercenary reasons, there are two motives of a higher sort, which undoubtedly exercise great influence on the choice of able and good men. The first is the *Scientific interest* of medical work. In this the profession stands almost alone, so as to become the natural vocation of a youth with scientific tastes. The second is the motive of pure *Humanity*, the simple desire to relieve the woes of suffering men and agonising women ; to diminish the pain of the world, and to prolong useful lives. This is a noble, a divine motive for the devotion of a life ; and it would be wrong to doubt that many a poor country practitioner, and many a skilful London physician, has been guided by this exalted feeling in his choice, just as truly as his brother has been led by genuine piety to enter the ministry of religion.

The fact, however, that there are many good men urged by none but the loftiest and purest motives, amid the thousands of whom the profession is composed, ought certainly not to make us leap to the conclusion that all doctors are pure enthusiasts of humanity. As an able writer in the *Spectator* well observed, it is as absurd to predicate the same moral character for all men who enter the medical profession as for all men who pass over West-minster Bridge. There are, as we have just seen, sufficient low motives, as well as high ones, to lead young men to such choice. It is the misfortune of the Clerical profession, that the performance of its ordinary duties requires an assump-tion of pious feeling which even sincerely religious men do not always hold ready at command. The consequence is (as Hume long ago explained) that genuinely good clergymen are often led into some sort of hollowness and affectation, while men who have entered the priesthood from merely secular motives are apt to degenerate into downright hypo-crites. In an analogous way, it is the misfortune of the

Medical profession that the performance of its ordinary
duties involves the appearance of humane feelings, which
may or may not be present on any particular occasion, but
which the patient and his friends usually expect to see
exhibited, and which the doctor is consequently almost
driven to simulate. Where the medical man is naturally
kind-hearted, there is no incongruity between his beneficent
act and benevolent sentiment, and no shade of hypocrisy
tarnishes his behaviour. But when the doctor has adopted
his profession as a mere *gagne-pain*, or from taste for science
rather than love of humanity, then a certain affectation of
sympathy with his patients and their afflicted friends is forced
upon him, and we behold the not very rare phenomenon of
a medical Tartuffe.

This matter is the more needful to be analysed, because
the idle ideas current about the "kindness" of doctors
make it seem, to not a few good souls, almost a sacrilege
to question any of the abuses of the profession. These
simple hearts totally forget that a patient is to a doctor
what a rock is to a geologist, or a flower to a botanist—the
much-coveted *subject of his studies*. If patients do not
come to a doctor, the doctor must go in search of patients;
and if he could not see them in the hospitals for nothing,
he would pay to be admitted to see them and exhibit them
to his pupils. Very often, when the sufferer or his friends
are with tearful gratitude thanking the doctor for having
remitted some portion of his fees, the learned man must
inwardly reflect that he would have paid a good round sum
rather than have missed so curious a case. Let any one try
(as the writer has done) to remove to better quarters a
pauper suffering from some "interesting" affliction, out of
the reach of a doctor who was attending him for "charity,"
and the sentiment of pure benevolence will not be so
manifest as might be expected. On the other hand, a
display of sympathy is part of the stock-in-trade of a

physician (especially of one who attends ladies), witnout which he could not hope for a large *clientèle*, any more than a grocer would succeed in business who failed in civility to his customers. Of course, there is much real, most disinterested kindness shown by medical men to their friends and patients. They would not be human if it were not so, and nobody dreams that they are insensible to the claims of charity or sympathy. But the everlasting "kindness" and "guinea-amiability," vouchsafed supremely to the wealthiest patients, is, as I have said, only part of the doctor's stock-in-trade, like the blue and red bottles in the chemist's shop.

Against the attractions of the medical profession now enumerated, sufficient to account for the adoption of it by so many thousands of youths, it is good to set the opposite circumstances, which deter from it a differently constituted order of minds. To begin with, few men of poetic temperament are likely, for very obvious reasons, to become doctors. To make the weaknesses and maladies of our poor human frames the subject of a whole life's study and attention, so that a man should, as it were, live evermore in a world of disease; to pass from one sick-room to another, and from a distressing sight to a fetid odour, in endless succession; to acquire knowledge by the dissection of corpses, and employ it, when gained, in amputating limbs, delivering women in childbirth, dressing sores, and inspecting everything ugly and loathsome to the natural senses,—this is surely a vocation which calls for either great enthusiasm or great callousness. The Doctor is, in truth, at the very antipodes from the Poet or the Artist. It would seem to outsiders as if a year of his profession would suffice to blot from the mind all the beauty of the world, and to spoil the charm and sanctity of the sweetest mysteries of human nature. Everything which the painter, the sculptor, the poet touches with reverent and loving hands—the soul-

speaking eye, the heaving breast, the lip which meets lip
in supremest emotion,—all these are to the doctor the seats
of so many diseases ; organs where he may look for an
amaurosis or a cancer. Of course, we know that men of
great refinement of feeling are found to conquer all such
natural repugnance, and suffering humanity may be grateful
(so far as medical science brings it relief) that there are
those who can do so, and even find the wards of a hospital
quite as delightful, and much more interesting, than the
terraces of a garden or the galleries of the Vatican. To
these æsthetic objections to the profession of medicine must
be added another of a different but scarcely less effectual
kind. Custom has settled that the mode of remuneration
for the services of doctors (in the higher walks especially)
should take the peculiarly awkward form of a direct transfer
of coin from the hand of the private patient. This practice,
even among well-bred persons, is liable to involve disagree-
able incidents, and with vulgar and rude ones must cause to
a physician of high spirit endless annoyances which are
wholly escaped in those professions wherein service is paid
by public salary or by fees which pass through an office.

We have seen who are our doctors, and why they choose
their profession. Next we may note, in passing, as regards
their education, that they commonly change in the tran-
sition from a medical Student to a full-blown Physician or
Surgeon, in a manner quite unparalleled by other youngsters.
The embryo parson, soldier, or lawyer, at Oxford or Sand-
hurst, or while "eating his dinners," is, indeed, usually a
little less sedate than he becomes a few years later ; but he
only differs from his adult self as the colt differs from the
horse, the playful puppy from the responsible mastiff. The
medical student, on the contrary, undergoes a transforma-
tion like that of a larva, when it becomes a moth. One day
we notice Bob Sawyer, as a rowdy and dissipated youth,
with linen of questionable purity, and a pipe and foul

language alternately in his mouth; the *bête-noire* of every modest girl, and the unfailing nuisance of every public meeting, where he may stamp and crow and misbehave himself. Anon, Robert Sawyer, Esq., M.D., or M.R.C.S., emerges the pink of cleanliness and decorum, to flit evermore softly through shaded boudoirs, murmuring soothing suggestions to ladies suffering from headaches, and recommending mild syrups to teething infants. His old celebrated canticle—

> Hurrah for the Cholera Morbus,
> Which brings us a guinea a-day,

has unaccountably been changed for such burning zeal to save humanity from disease, that he is ready to persecute anti-vaccinators to the death, or cut up any number of living dogs and cats merely on the chance of discovering some remedy for human suffering.[*]

We now reach the most important feature of the subject, the general Moral Character of the profession; and here we must all thankfully recognise that medical men, as a body (after their studentship), exhibit many virtues, and comparatively few of the grosser vices. So far as the memory of the present writer extends, there have been no worse or more numerous scandals affecting doctors during the last twenty years, than affecting the clergy.

[*] The late Dr. Carpenter (*Modern Review.* July, 1881. p. 499) says that the above passage "bespeaks either gross ignorance or malicious fooling. No modest girl has now anything more to fear from Medical students than from the undergraduates of our Universities." In reply to this it might be enough to refer to the Police Reports generally; but it will be better to quote the *Medical Times'* opinion of the project of opening a suitable residence with supervision for Medical students in London. "We would much rather see the London Medical student as he is, a *little wild*, a *little rough* and *guilty perhaps of occasional lapses from virtue*, than have him surrounded by the refined fripperies and the polished restraint of an academic life. More billiards if you like; but, Proctors, distinctly No! . . . . Make the student more *virtuous* and *you will make the practitioner more vicious.*"—*Medical Times,* November 1, 1884. (Italics ours.)

They are industrious when poor, and often 'liberal when rich. In times of war, or epidemics, their devotion to their chosen tasks rises, not seldom, to true heroism. The ordinary English country practitioner, with his small pay, his rough work in all weathers, and his general kindliness and honesty, is one of the most respectable and valuable members of the community. This and more may be said to the credit of the profession. On the other side there are grave charges and suspicions (chiefly attaching to the fashionable physicians and surgeons of the great cities and health resorts), which, though not often openly expressed or marshalled together, are yet sown broadcast through the minds of the laity, and which it is highly desirable should be fairly stated, and then either rejected as unjust, or allowed their due weight in the guidance of conduct between the public and the profession.

It would be exceedingly unjust to include among the elements of such a judgment as this the exceptional crimes—murders, adulteries, and seductions—which may be laid to the charge of individual offenders in every profession. The only point regarding these which here concerns us is the obvious fact that, if by any misfortune a man with criminal proclivities enters the medical profession, he possesses, as a doctor, unparalleled facilities for the commission and concealment of crime. A Prichard or a La Pommeray, handsome and gentlemanly, who may desire to remove a rich wife or mistress out of the way, either to inherit her money or marry another woman, can scarcely find any difficulty in administering a slow poison, or so arranging things as that the victim shall swallow a rapid one by mistake. Even the purchase and possession of deadly drugs (in other men a damning evidence of guilt), scarcely afford ground of suspicion against a doctor. Of course, we know that not one doctor in 500 can for a moment be suspected of such crimes ; but who will venture to say that not one in 5,000, or one in 25,000, doctors may prove another Palmer or Webster or Prichard, or such a reckless wretch as he who, a few years ago, answered the advertisement offering £60 for a poison?

It is a serious question whether, in the event of the commission of such crimes, we should find medical coroners alert and firm in dragging to light every suspicious circumstance and sending the case unhesitatingly to trial, or whether they would let down their colleague as easily as might be practicable, and direct their jury to find a verdict of "Misadventure." The same remarks apply to crimes of another cast—seduction, adultery, and offences committed on narcotised victims. Doctors are as little open to such charges as other men, but not *less* so; and again it must be borne in mind that they meet temptations and possess facilities for committing and concealing such offences which fall to no other lot.

Leaving now this question of exceptional crimes, which ought to be excluded from our judgment of the general character of the profession, let us inquire, first, what are the principles supposed to prevail amongst medical men? and then, secondly, what can we gleam concerning their practice?

It has been long generally believed that while the profession on the Continent is almost to a man, Atheist, a milder and less defined Materialism is usually accepted by English medical men as their philosophy of the universe. Of late years the homage paid by the profession to certain eminent men of science has, rightly or wrongly, conveyed the impression that nine doctors out of ten, if they spoke out, would call themselves Agnostics. * These gentlemen may perhaps say that it is no business of their patients to ask what are their private opinions on theology and morals so

---

* So far as we can learn, doctors in country parishes mostly profess Church principles, and, occasionally, go to Church. In London they send their wives, to represent them.

long as they administer to them the right drugs and set their
bones, *secundum artem*. But, in truth, it *is* the business of
everybody to learn what are the genuine beliefs of men who
are certain ere long to leaven society therewithal. The
doctors are now much more to us than drug administrators
and bone-setters. Few prospects are more profoundly
alarming than the advance to ubiquitous influence of an order
of men who should, as a rule, reject and despise those ultimate
faiths of the human heart in God and Duty and Immortality, which ennoble and purify mortal life as no physiological science can ennoble, and no physical "sanitation"
purify. It is a matter of importance to every individual
amongst us to know whether the man who will stand by
our death-bed and the death-beds of our beloved ones, will
help us to look up beyond the gaping grave, or will throw the
pall of his silence and disbelief over the flickering flame of
dying hope and prayer.

There are missionary physicians now sent forth into
many heathen countries (notably to Japan), where they
effect more conversions than all the clerical missionaries
together. Who can help foreseeing that the converse will
happen at home, if the doctors who come closest to every
man and woman in the supreme hours of life and death
should exhale their dead and hopeless materialism in every
word and look? The man who entertains a private
conviction that the tender emotions are merely glandular
"affections," and that a mother's love, a poet's inspira-
tion, a saint's prayer, are simply transformed beef and
mutton, bread and beer—this man must, even if he be
never so reticent, draw a trail of cold and slimy doubt over
the fairest and noblest things in human life. There is, of
course, a great and ever-present temptation to a physician
to view things from the material, or (as our fathers would
have called it) the carnal side ; to think always of the
influence of the body on the mind, rather than of the mind

on the body; to place the interests of Health in the van, and those of Duty in the rear; to study physiological rather than psychological phenomena; nay, to centre attention on the morbid phases of both bodily and mental conditions rather than on the normal and healthful ones of the *mens sana in corpore sano.* All the more reason, then, is there anxiously to desire that the man subjected to such downward pressure should possess some faith on whose wings he may be lifted above the mire. Woe to him, and to all whom he may influence, when a doctor is at once in theory and practice, a Materialist and a Disease-monger.*

Be the principles and opinions of the medical profession what they may, we have now to consider their practical conduct. The observations to be made on this matter may fall under five heads.

1. The *raison d'être* of the medical profession is to cure the diseases, relieve the pains, and, when possible, prolong the lives of men. To attain these beneficent ends, Science must be the guide—Anatomical Science, Physiological Science, Chemical Science, and so on. Honour is justly due, then, to the physician who *studies science in order to cure his patients.*

But is it equally honourable to *study patients in order to acquire science?* Is it well to treat suffering human beings, —as, in the medical jargon of the day,—merely so much "*clinical material?*" Is it right to consider hospitals as primarily existing, not that patients may be cured, but that doctors may be trained? Assuredly, whether it be, or be not, morally justifiable to look on men and women in such a light, it is not to do so that *doctors are*

* There exists a Medical Ritualistic Brotherhood, styled the Guild of S. Luke. Hopes were entertained at its formation that it would set itself to oppose the abuses of the profession; but they have been regretfully abandoned since the publication, in *Macmillan's Magazine*, of a paper by the secretary, defending Vivisection with the usual base appeal to human selfishness and cowardice.

paid, either by their private patients or by the public which supports the hospitals. The impression may be false, and is necessarily vague, but it is extremely strong and widespread that the primary beneficent object of the profession, its only ostensible object—namely, Healing—is daily more and more subordinated to the secondary object, namely, Scientific Investigation ; in short, that the means have become the end, and the end the means It is believed that patients having diseases scientifically interesting, are needlessly detained in hospitals, and, instead of being treated with a single-eyed view to restoration to health, are subjected to experiments calculated to elucidate pathological problems even at the cost of prolonged suffering or increased danger.*

* In a letter in the *Times*, dated November 22, 1883, a London physician of high standing, Dr. Watteville, after rebuking another person for bringing a charge against a doctor "of having used patients in a hospital for other purposes than those tending to their own direct benefit," proceeds to say : "So far from there being a reason why moral and pecuniary support should be refused to hospitals on the ground *that their inmates are made use of otherwise than for treatment*, there is even ground why more should be given to them in order to compensate by every possible comfort for the *discomforts necessarily entailed by the education of succeeding generations of medical men*, &c." "Sentimentalists who uphold the abstract rights of men and want to push them to their logical consequences have no other alternative in the question now before us than *to condemn the modern course of medical studies*." The reader will likewise remember the exposure of the experiments on Hospital patients by Drs. Ringer and Murrell in 1883. Commenting upon them, the *Standard*, November 1, said : "It is beyond controversy that nitrite of sodium was administered to 47 patients, producing in the large majority of cases the most distressing effects, not, apparently, to the surprise of the medical men who were conducting these observations. One at least of these 47 patients had nothing the matter with him except 'a little rheumatism.' What the others were suffering from we do not know." . . . . In a letter signed "M.D.," also in the *Standard* at the same time, the writer quotes Dr. Ringer's "Handbook of Therapeutics," 8th edition, p. 340, where it appears that the author and three other doctors cited had given twelve ounces of good brandy to one man in a single dose, making him "dead drunk," to "healthy young men" other huge quantities ; and on "*a boy aged ten who had never in his life before taken alcohol in any form*," they made a "large number of observations" of the same kind, apparently to settle some problem about reduction of temperature.

Similarly, in private houses, if experimentation be rare, the physician yet often betrays that his interest centres on the purely scientific aspect of the case. He gives himself great pains to make "an accurate diagnosis," to be verified, perhaps, hereafter, by a "successful post-mortem ;" but of the means of *cure* he thinks so little that he has been sometimes observed to start, when asked by the not-unreasonably vexed patient, what he recommends him to do? and to reply, "Oh, to be sure! you ought to do something; I will write a prescription." By-and-by, patients will begin to recalcitrate at paying heavily to afford their doctor another "case" to classify in the tables of his learned work on the lungs, the liver, or the brain, whereon he expects to found his claim to immortality and profit. They will say with Pliny, "Discunt periculis nostris et per experientiam mortem agunt."*

Nor is it only for the sake of acquiring knowledge, but also for that of imparting it, that medical men are believed to sacrifice their patients' interests. The poor sufferers who accept the charity of the public hospitals do so on the condition of allowing the students, as well as the doctors, to inspect their cases. But it is plain as daylight that this condition becomes morally abrogated when the patient's recovery would be postponed or imperilled by the distressing circumstances of exposure and bedside lecturing. Such limitation, however, is rarely, if ever, regarded, and decent women, afflicted with some of the most dreadful diseases of humanity, find, in these so-called charitable institutions,

---

* Dr. Burney Yeo, writing in the *Medical Times*, May 17, 1884, contrasted the Regular Physician with those Irregular people who only aim at curing disease. "How different," he remarks, "is the aim of the physician! He works not for the one, but for the many; not for the individual, but for humanity!" May we not reasonably ask, whether the "one," the "individual,' who *pays* the physician the fee for this large-aimed work, is quite aware that *his* recovery is not the aim of his adviser, but rather the benefit of humanity on the whole by the advancement of science *at his expense?*

moral tortures of outraged modesty added to their bodily anguish. No doctor can be dull enough to ignore the fact that the feelings of a woman with a crowd of curious young students round her bed of agony, must be almost worse than death, and must lessen her chances of recovery, if any such there be. But when does one of these teachers and guides of youth spare the shame-tortured woman at the cost of Mr. Bob Sawyer's disappointment?

Again, patients are sacrificed not merely at the shrine of knowledge, but on the anvil of manipulative skill. That operations are performed for the sake either of acquiring such skill, or keeping the surgeon's hand well "in"—as well as of earning enormous fees—we have the best evidence. The late eminent and honest surgeon, Mr. Skey, openly denounced this abuse, and said, "A man who has the reputation of a splendid operator is ever a just object of suspicion." Probably every reader will recollect cases where a leg or arm has been amputated, and after a time it was found that the frightful sacrifice might have been spared. These are the men who, as Tennyson says, are

Happier in using the knife than in trying to save the limb.

When we think of the cruelty—as bad as that of any tyrant of old—of reducing a man or women to the miserable condition of a one-armed or one-legged creature, or of rendering a young wife for ever excluded from the joys of motherhood, and of the selfishness which can make a surgeon, for the sake of either his skill or his fee, recommend an operation which might have been avoided, we have some measure of the hardness of heart which is at least *possible* in the profession, according to the testimony of one of its most honoured members. Let anyone who questions the truth of these

A pair of the most beautiful eyes known to the writer were only preserved in the handsome head to which they belong, by the refusal of the young owner to profit by the urgent recommendation of one of the first oculists of the day to allow him to relieve her of one splendid orb at the moderate cost, perhaps,

remarks examine the correspondence and leading articles thereon which appeared in the *Liverpool Courier*, for August and September, 1886, concerning the 111 operations on women performed in **the Shaw Street** Hospital during the previous year. **The *Lancet*, speaking of the trial of** one of **the doctors concerned (prosecuted by the indignant husband** of one of **the patients), remarked, " The interest of the trial** lies in the **question whether the frequent and almost indis**criminate **use "** of the awful operation in **question, on women** *"suffering from diseases which are* **not fatal and are** *often only trivial,* is justifiable **?** The highest authorities in this country have justly condemned the frequent performance of this operation "—(ovariotomy).

And here we must recall to those who forget **it,** that this recklessness and pitilessness of doctors was betrayed forty years ago, when they permitted Burke and Hare to bring **them corpses for anatomical study,** which were well-nigh unmistakably those **of foully murdered men. If** *this* were possible among those to **whom the " Burkers "** brought their victims, it is idle **to doubt that others may** amputate limbs which might be saved, or detain interesting "cases" **for** years on beds of pain,—all in " the sacred interests **of science."**

2. It is not only for the sake of science that **the interests** of patients are believed to be sacrificed by **medical men.** The pecuniary interests, either of individual **doctors or of** the profession at large, seem to outweigh such **considerations** in numberless cases.* To take a simple example. What are

* Here is what one of the organs of the profession, with **refreshing frankness** not to say cynicism, says on this head, discussing **the question of Notification** of Diseases :—" Let us not pretend to more virtue **for medical men than for** other classes of practitioners of similar social standing ; and let us, therefore, **not forget that a** very **numerous section of** our profession **will certainly not** if they can help it, do **anything which will** interfere with their own interests or practice. With such **practitioners business is business.** If the notification fee is half-a-crown, they will notify for **the purpose of earning it ; but if it** pays them sixpence more **to pretend not to recognise** a case of infectious disease, they certainly will **be very slow to find out what in reality is wrong** with the patient."—*Medical* **Press and Circular,** January 10, 1883.

the motives of those luminaries who recommend all the bad
wines and sickly beverages which we see advertised every
day in the newspapers? A more certain way of promoting
disease than the recommendation of some of this rubbish
is scarcely conceivable. A famous American surgeon was
offered £1,000 to puff one of these drinks (by no means the
worst) and act as its usher to the New York market. This
doctor, being honest, declined the bribe. Are we to consider
that others do not entertain similar scruples?

The same question may be asked respecting all the
remedies which by turns come into fashion. We look
back with amused disgust at what doctors have done in
times past in the way of recommending useless and noxious
nostrums one after another; but we forget that they are
always at the same tricks, and that every year sees some
new and costly *fad* of medicine solemnly adopted by all the
lights of the profession, as surely as a new cut in dresses is
adopted by the milliners; and just as certainly next year
quietly dropped into oblivion.

The reckless multiplication of expensive prescriptions is
another "bone" which patients with limited means may
well pick with their doctors. Did any one ever rally from
an illness, or clear a room after a death, without finding at
least twenty half-used bottles of draughts and embrocations
and gargles, and as many boxes of pills on the table? The
entente cordiale between the physician and the chemist, and
perhaps certain percentages, are not unconnected with these
"untasted relics of the feast."

A much more serious matter, however, is the question,
How far do medical men generally really and honestly
strive to cure their well-paying patients? How far do they
deceive them about their ailments, and give them advice
which, instead of restoring them to health and vigour, is
calculated to keep them on the sick list? Medicine can, at
best, not do much; some of us think it can do very little,

and the great new sect of " Natural Doctors " in Germany
are beginning to show cause for trusting nature to herself
alone, without drugs or blisters or phlebotomy, merely
securing for her the best conditions of quiet and air,
warmth or coolness, at our disposal. But assuming that
medicines can really cure disease, how painful is the doubt
whether the doctor whom we employ to use them for our
benefit may turn them to our hurt! To be robbed by the
policeman, or to have our premises burnt down by the
watchman, is a small vexation compared to being kept ill
by the man we pay to make us well. But does this disaster
never befall us, though, perhaps, we rarely recognise the
humiliating fact? We have all read the mutual accusations
of making business for themselves, which the lawyers have
been bandying about; and we remember the good story of
the old solicitor who received with horror from his son and
partner (left in charge of his office during a trip abroad) the
intelligence that the foolish young man had brought to a
sudden conclusion a great Chancery suit which had provided
an income for the family for ten years back, and might have
done the same for ten years more. Similar grim jokes concern every profession and every trade. The difference in
their application to the medical profession is, that much
closer interests are involved, and the fraud practised is infinitely more cruel.

Let us consider what are the *presumptions* against the
doctors, since of actual evidence, from the nature of the
case, there can be little. Let it be granted that in cases
of febrile and acute diseases there is reason to hope
that they do their best to effect a cure. What of other and
chronic diseases? What of the worst of all,—Lunacy. for
example? Does the mad-doctor of the private asylum, who
makes £200 or £300 a year by a wealthy patient, really lay
himself out, with all his skill, to heal the poor bewildered
brain? Does he never allow the patient to excite him-

self before the visitors, so as to bring on accesses of his disorder, and confirm the belief that he still requires incarceration when he might be set at liberty? A clear-sighted author talks of " unconscious bias produced by pecuniary interests ; " and, truly, human nature being what it is, nobody can think it otherwise than a mis-fortune that the interest of a physician in cases of such extreme doubt and delicacy should always be on one side, and the recovery of the patient on the other. The Press has pronounced again and again that lunatics ought only to be confined in public asylums, where the physicians should receive fixed salaries, and a *bonus on recoveries,*—not payment by the case. By such judgments they have tacitly avowed the belief that this most grievous of the woes of humanity is left, by the cupidity of the doctors, to press on many a soul from which it might be lifted off. To quote the direct evidence on the subject would involve endless controversy. It is well known 'to all interested in the subject.

And what of other chronic diseases—neuralgia, and gout, and heart-disease, and headaches, and all the nameless woes of rich and feminine mortality? We laugh at the legend of the physicians of the Chinese Emperor, whose salaries are stopped when their celestial patron is ill, and only run again when he is restored to health. But though we cannot copy this ingenious plan from the Flowery Land, we most of us believe that out of our twenty thousand doctors there are not a few (and they, *by the hypothesis,* among the wealthy and prosperous) who are far from insensible to the tempta-tion of keeping a well-paying patient for months and years in a state of valetudinarianism. When we see a peevish old man always in the gout, or a fine lady always stretched on her sofa smelling *eau-de-Cologne*, we may safely look out of window for the carriage of the unctuous doctor, whose yearly income would be considerably lessened by the restoration of the gentleman to the moors, and of the lady to the duties of her household and nursery. If we ask one of these poor medical *pièces de résistance* why he or she does not at least try fresh air, or riding exercise, or Turkish baths, it is singular how invariably they have been told by dear Dr. Hushaby that any such efforts would involve deadly danger to their "hearts."*

A medical treatise, intended only for the profession, contains these significant words :—"*If* cure be an object in the case, then " so-and-so is to be done. Apparently there are cases where cure is not an object ! Plumbers are popularly believed never to mend one hole in the leads of a house without making another. The gentlemen whom we call in to tinker our internal pipes and gutters, it is to be feared sometimes adopt similar tactics. Let us suppose a true specific remedy found for gout, neuralgia, or dyspepsia, which, by cheap and easy private application, would make every patient suffering from those diseases as sound as a trivet. What welcome would that blessed remedy receive from the medical Profession? When the news of its existence became irrepressible, how many rich patients would be assured that, for their particular case, a trial of it might entail fatal consequences ?

These terrible charges have not only been made by outsiders and satirists from Molière downwards, but have been repeated with fitting grief and indignation quite recently by honest and honourable members of the profession itself, proving that they by no means concern only a past order of things. Here is what Dr. Russell Reynolds, F.R.S., said in 1881, in an address to the Medical Society of University

* To the personal knowledge of the present writer, three ladies, after periods varying from six to fourteen years of the sofa, were roused to break their silken chains, and suddenly found they could get up and live like other people. In one case the poor dame, having renounced her doctor and all his ordinances, after long childlessness, became the joyful mother of a healthy little babe.

College (to the Hospital of which College he is Consulting Physician), and which address was published at the time in the *British Medical Journal* :—

"There is meddling and muddling of a most disreputable sort, and the patients" (he is speaking of women) "grow sick of it and give it all up and get well; or they go from bad to worse." . . . . "Physicians have coined names for trifling maladies if they have not invented them and have set fashions of disease. They have treated or maltreated their patients by endless examinations, applications, and the like, and this sometimes for months, sometimes for years, and then, when by some accident the patient has been removed from their care, she has become quite well and there has been no more need for caustic," &c., &c.

And here is a still more horrible accusation in the same Address against those doctors whose specialism is the diseases of men.

"Are there not some who prey upon the sense of shame and extort money for needless operations and worthless drugs, holding in terror over their victims the knowledge of facts that have been confided to them? The consulting room—as sacred as the confessional—is degraded to the lowest depths of degradation when it is used or abused as the engine of terror or extortion. But yet bills are incurred and bills are drawn and Jews are sought for in order to meet the so-called obligations of these sufferers. The surgeon has the power in his hand, and he knows it, and wields it often with a cruelty which no words of mine can utter or sufficiently condemn."—*British Medical Journal*, Oct. 15th, 1881, p. 621.

And here is what Dr. Clifford Allbut said, in delivering the Gulstonian Lecture for 1884, at the Royal College of Physicians. After referring with compassion to the sufferings of women, who, he believes, "feel pain more than men do," he mentioned the "*morbid chains*," the "*mental abase-*

ment" into which fall "the flock of women who lie under
the wand of the Gynæcologist" (specialist of women's diseases) ; "*the women who are caged up in London back
drawing-rooms, and visited almost daily*, their brave and
active spirits broken under a false (! !) belief in the presence
of a secret and over-mastering local malady ; and the best
years of their lives honoured only by a distressful victory
over pain." (Italics ours.)—*Medical Press*, March 19, 1884.

3. Beside these matters, wherein the individual doctor's
profits are in one scale and the patient's in another, there
is a still more important class of cases, wherein the interests
of the profession are on one side and those of the public on
the other. In these latter there is reason to apprehend that
a tacit trades-unionism exists among all medical men,
whereby the interests of the laity are systematically sacrificed to those of the profession.

As a first example of this trades-unionism, let us take the
case of Consultations of doctors, wherein it is obvious that
some well-understood bye-law forbids the physician called
in consultation to allow a suspicion to go abroad that his
colleague, originally in charge of the case, has made a blunder
and brought the patient to death's door. Proverbially,
"doctors differ," and agreement under other circumstances
is so rare that it may be dismissed from calculation. But
let great Dr. A., from London, be summoned to Cornwall
or Northumberland to consult with Dr. B., a country
practitioner of respectable standing, about a case of im-
minent peril, and what becomes of the proverbial "differ
ence"? Dr. A., with a solemnity which must tax his
gravity and that of his colleague like the meeting of two
augurs of old, assures the heart-broken mother, or wife soon
to be a widow, that "everything has been done in the very
best and wisest way possible, that the patient could not be
in better hands than those of Dr. B.," and, finally (as if to
save the appearance of utter inutility of the costly visit), that

"the patient may now take a second tablespoonful of the same mixture as before." When this solemn farce has been played, Dr. A., who has eaten an excellent luncheon in the house of mourning, presses the hand of the miserable wife, pockets his magnificent fee, steps into the carriage waiting to carry him back to the station, and reads on his way up to town a charming article on that intense sympathy of medical men for suffering humanity which "makes them ready to sacrifice hecatombs of brutes to save the smallest pain of a man."

What has that smooth-spoken doctor done? In the sight of God he has told a shameful and cruel lie, and has taken money from the very victim of his falsehood. He has betrayed the trust of loving and simple hearts, and left them to break, when with a word he might have done what in him lay to save their earthly treasure.

If doctors will do this cruel and wicked thing for their trades-union, what will they *not* do likewise? And who amongst the readers of this paper can recall any case where they have acted otherwise, and spoken the truth; except when the doctor, perhaps, whose patient they visited, happened to be of so humble a class, that the great man could venture to treat him as he pleased? *

Let us, for heaven's sake, know where we stand. Will the doctors tell us truth beside the sick-beds of our friends,

---

* An Instructive episode, throwing light on the matter, is that of Sir William Gull's evidence on a trial, some years ago, of a Guy's Hospital nurse. The Court asked Sir William Gull, "In your opinion, should a skilful physician have known that brain disease existed?" Sir William replied, "There I must be careful. There is, no doubt, great difficulty in recognising brain disease at that stage . . . but I cannot doubt that suspicion ought to have existed." Later on, he refused to say, though pressed by Dr. Pavy's counsel, that suspicion was very often incorrect. For this breach of medical etiquette, Sir William Gull, a man at the very summit of the profession, was actually complained against by Dr. Pavy (the physician who might have entertained the "suspicions") before the College of Physicians, and the President and Censors, having solemnly deliberated on the matter, pronounced judgment on the 12th January, 1881, to the following effect : That they "do not deem the

or will they *not!* If they will not, then let us be relieved from the monstrous cost and heart-breaking disappointments consequent on summoning them to consultations.

This question of the secret understanding and trades-union bye-laws among medical men rises to the level of political importance when we note that our coroners are now so generally taken from the profession. The particular duty of a coroner and his jury in scores of cases is to deal with charges directly concerning doctors, and to decide whether they have administered wrong medicines, or connived at child-murder before or after birth, or neglected to attend to a dying pauper patient, or discharged a patient from a hospital who ought to have been retained, or vaccinated in such a manner as to entail death. It is essential we should know what are the rules of behaviour for a medical coroner under such circumstances according to medical morality. What will his professional conscience require him to do as regards his colleague? Is he to act simply as an honest coroner in the interest of the public, drag every case fully to light, and send such as seem to deserve it to trial? Or is he to screen his medical brother by every available artifice and all the influence over the jury at his command, and never let any scandal come to light or any case go into court which he can by any means smother and suppress?

Reference to another evidence of the extent of the trade-

character of the evidence which a member of the College has given on oath in a Court of Justice a proper subject to investigate when the Court has expressed itself satisfied in regard to the truthfulness and sincerity of the witness," &c.

In reviewing this decision, which, truly to the non-medical mind, appears a matter of course (the converse sentence being inconceivable), the *British Medical Journal* (Jan. 29, p. 167), says—" The evidence given upon oath in such cases is in the highest degree privileged . . . But it must be a very delicate matter for a chartered body, such as the College of Physicians, having certain powers entrusted by law to its Board of Censors, to deal with a complaint against evidence given upon oath by one of its fellows in a Court of Law." Very "delicate" indeed! But what if the evidence were not "privileged," and only given at the bedside of a dying man, in return for a fee of a hundred guineas?

unionism among medical men has been already made in speaking of the unanimity wherewith the profession as a body, having itself very little concern with Vivisection, has supported the handful of physiologists in their demand for a "free vivisecting table." The memorial against Lord Carnarvon's Bill, presented to the Home Office, on the 10th July, 1876, was signed by 3,000 medical men, and presented by such a crowd as never before invaded a Ministerial office, except, perhaps, in a revolution; and all this excitement was drawn forth at a moment's notice.* Previous to the manipulation of their wire-pullers there were numerous medical men ready to denounce the abuses of the practice. Sixty of them at first signed the original Memorial to the Jermyn Street Society, and before the Royal Commission, eighteen of them gave the opinion that the practice ought to be placed under legislative restraint. The Bill introduced by their ordinary Parliamentary representative, Dr. Lyon Playfair, was entirely in the same spirit. But the stupid cry was raised that any restriction on the cutting up of live animals would be an affront to their profession (which had very cheerfully submitted to a similar restriction in cutting up dead men!), and from that moment there has been a closing of the ranks, from which only a few brave and self-respecting men have had the courage to come forth.

The Vaccination controversy is one on which it would be idle here to enter; but if the reader bear in mind the fact that between 1840 and 1886 the doctors received £2,508,237 out of the rates for vaccination, independently of private practice † (See Reports of Local Government Board), the

* For a full account of the attitude of the Medical Profession on this subject, see a paper by Miss Frances Power Cobbe in the *Contemporary Review*, "Mr. Lowe and the Vivisection Act," reprinted by the Victoria Street Society.

† How great the value of this private practice of Vaccination must be may be guessed from the fact that on the occasion of a panic at Eton some years

zealotry and cruelty wherewith this medical "rite" is upheld, will scarcely escape the suspicion of the before-named "unconscious bias produced by pecuniary interest." Baptism was never urged by those who believed that it could save Souls from perdition, with such relentlessness as Vaccination is insisted upon by men whose "cardinal doctrine," as Mr. Shorter says, "is Salvation by Filth," and who insist that it can save Bodies from small-pox.*

Considering the success of Jenner's discovery (indisputabie, at all events, so far as affording business to doctors is concerned), it is not astonishing that Pasteur's similar, but exceedingly cruel, invention should have been hailed with rapture by the mouthpieces of the profession. The prospect of Pasteur Institutes rising up on all sides, each with its well-paid staff of inoculators and vivisectors, has seemed infinitely more attractive than .the simple and inexpensive Buisson treatment of hydrophobia by Vapour baths ; albeit, the latter has been known to cure the actually-developed disease, while Pasteur already counts more than 40 deaths as the upshot of his "preventive" measures.

ago, a single doctor pocketed £400 for vaccinating 800 scholars. Is it wonderful that we should read in the *British Medical Journal* (Oct. 23, 1886) such sentences as the following: "Dr. Bruce Low is of opinion that some system of compulsory re-vaccination should he adopted to protect the nation —and suggests that all children leaving school should bo re-vacoinatod at the public cost"?

* The trades-unionism, which commands at once the doctors who register deaths, tho doctors who profit by compulsory vaccination, and the coroners who direct the juries in cases of alleged death from vaccination, is amusingly illustrated by such facts as the following, nooted by Mr Peter Taylor in Parliament: Mr. Henry Hay, Health Officer to the Aston Juion, birmingham, writes: "A death from the first cause (erysipelas after vaccination) occurred not long ago in my practice, and although I had not vaccinated the child, yet in my desire to *preserve vaccination from reproach*, I omitted all mention of it in my certificate of death." Again, tho value of a medical coroner was exemplified at Leeds, where an inquest was held on a child who had died of the results of vaccination. The coroner declined to accept that statement as a verdict, and told the jury "there was no such thing known to the law as death from vaccination," and they must bring in "died by the visitation of God."

Beyond the demand for unrestricted Vivisection, and for compulsory Vaccination, and re-vaccination, we now hear (1886) that the public will be taxed, if the doctors can manage it, to support an enormous corps of dentists who are to have the supervision of all the teeth of all the children in " all the public schools " of England, including the Reformatories and Training-Ships. Such at least is the programme of Mr. Fisher, read with great applause at the recent meeting of the British Dental Association at Dundee. Dr. Alderson goes further, and, as President of the West London Chirurgical Society, advocated at its Meeting, Oct. 8, 1886, " the principle of ' Health Assurance,' *i.e.*, the practice of paying medical men annually, ill or well, a certain fixed payment "—" the appointment of pathologists in every district, and, likewise, of School Visitors and School Board Examiners, from the ranks of medicine."—*Lancet.* Oct. 30.

All this, however, is of small account compared to another matter whereupon difference of opinion exists among medical men, and a few of them have honourably distinguished themselves by denouncing the abominable oppression. As a *profession*, however, the guilt and shame of the atrocious Contagious Diseases Acts lie at the door of the medical men of England, and it is their gross materialism, their utter disregard for human souls when lodged in the bodies of the despised and wretched, which made such legislation possible, and supported it for long years till the conscience of the lay public swept it away in disgust.

4. And now let us turn away from this last and darkest charge against medical men, and ask what truth there may be in the boast that they are the best friends of women, and that women may rightly trust them with grateful and unhesitating confidence? To the *fallen* we have seen they have gone out of their way to add a yet deeper degradation to their miserable fate; nor may they

boast that they can set against this any effort on their part
to extend relief or comfort of any sort to well-conducted
women of the working classes. It has been left for a woman-
doctor (Dr. Frances Hoggan) publicly to claim, though
not yet, alas! to obtain, for such humble women their
rightful share of the rates in the erection of resting-places
for themselves and their young children as they traverse
London. The male doctors have known all the sufferings
and disease entailed on poor mothers by the lack of such
temporary shelters, yet never have troubled themselves to
say one word on the subject. Such are the doctors to
women of the humbler classes. What are they to ladies?
Undoubtedly they know their interests too well to fail to
ingratiate themselves with them. But for real help what
have they to show? Did they ever make any serious effort
to stop the senseless and health-destroying fashion of
women's dress, the reckless dissipation and late hours which
have sent thousands of thoughtless girls to their graves?
A few Eli-like words of mild advice was all they ever uttered
against these deadly and wicked follies.

The case was reversed, however, when there was a move-
ment for the Higher Education of women, and it became
obvious that one of the aims of that education would be
to fit lady doctors to enter the market as competitors with
the men who had hitherto monopolised the profits of the
profession. Then, indeed, the doctors grew earnest and
made a grand discovery—namely, that mental labour is
peculiarly injurious to the weaker sex—much worse, it
would appear, for their feeble constitutions, than any
amount of ball-going and dissipation ; and that, in short,
a term at Girton was worse than five London seasons.
Women would perish, and the human race cease to mul-
tiply, if female intellects ascended from gossip to Greek
This spectre is nearly laid after ten years' exorcism, but
women cannot forget to what order of men they owe its

humiliating introduction ; and, Dr. Withers Moore has
this year (1886) taken pains to revive their memory of the
fact.

But, in spite of these solemn warnings, the ladies' insisted
on reading both Greek and Latin, and eke all the learned
treatises on anatomy and physiology and chemistry wherewith the intellects of doctors are supposed to be as full as
is a doll of bran. Then came the tug of war! Should
ladies be admitted, first to medical tuition and then to
medical degrees, and licence to practise? The remem-
brance is fresh in all our minds of the struggle in Edin-
burgh and elsewhere, and the chivalrous conduct of the
doctors and medical students on the occasion. Never,
indeed, has there been a more absurd public manifestation
of trades-unionism than this effort to keep ladies out of the
lucrative profession of physicians, and crowd them into
ill-paid one of nurses—for which (they were assured with
the most eager iteration) they were specially and solely
qualified.* At last Nemesis sent a bevy of lady nurses to
Guy's Hospital; and the doctors will probably henceforward
find reasons why they should no more be nurses than
physicians.

5. We pass lastly to the outlook for the public in future
years supposing the ambition of the medical profession to
proceed at its present rate of growth for another half-cen-
tury. It is obvious that Acts of Parliament, of which the
Compulsory Vaccination Act and the Contagious Diseases
Acts are the preludes, will then be multiplied till it may be
hard to name the department of human existence—birth,
marriage, education, employment, sickness, or death—in
which a doctor's certificate, a doctor's attendance, in short,
a doctor's well-paid sanction, shall not have become impera-

* For a history of the long struggle of the lady doctors and the behaviour
of their opponents, see an article in the *Contemporary Review* by Right Hon.
James Stansfeld, M.P.

tive, and the power of the profession to intrude and trammel
and interfere and enforce its exactions rendered practically
boundless. As a single specimen of what is already con-
templated in this way, we need only refer to the horrible
proposal to compel parents, children, husbands, and wives to
submit to be separated from their beloved ones in cases
of infectious disease, and to send them to be treated at the
discretion of a medical man. The day when this atrocious
scheme is legalised. either in Switzerland (where it
made some progress through the Legislature), or here in
England, will be "the beginning of the end" of all family
happiness. Cowardice is always cruel, but the cruelty of
this proposal to tear asunder the holiest ties in the hour
when they ought to be closest drawn, is a surprising revela-
tion of the poltroonery to which we are advancing in our
abject terror of disease. Better would it be that pestilence
should rage through the land, and we should die of "the
visitation of God," than that we should seek safety by
the abandonment of our nearest and dearest in the hour of
mortal trial, and leave them to the tender mercies of the
men who could call on us for such a sacrifice of affection
and duty.*

Space forbids that we should proceed further now in
pointing out the many lines of legislative interference

* And while the laity are patiently listening to this vile project, the men
who propose it are themselves running about with the utmost carelessness
between infected and non-infected patients. Are doctors, forsooth, of different flesh and blood from other men that infection does not cling to them
and they cannot convey it, since no one thinks of them as the over-active
disseminators of zymotic diseases all over the country? They have never
been required (as they ought to be) to abandon one or other half of their
practice, and confine themselves either to infectious or non-infectious cases.
They are not even bound by any custom of their own to take the trouble to
go home and bathe or change their specially dangerous cloth clothes before
they pass from a small-pox patient's death-bed to the bedside of a woman
giving birth to a child! They must be asked for no such sacrifice of profit
or time! but they call on us to sacrifice what is infinitely more precious—our
fondest affections and the most sacred duties which Providence has laid on
us between the cradle and the grave.

which the medical profession is sure to try, and which it will behove the public to watch with closest jealousy. It must suffice if we have here succeeded in placing before the reader some solid grounds for accepting the following conclusions :—

1. That the proper beneficent objects of the medical profession are being supplanted by the ardour of purely scientific investigation.

2. That the pecuniary interests of the profession frequently override the interests of patients.

3. That a trades-unionism exists in the profession which militates against the proper performance of the duties of medical men in various public and private offices.

4. That the profession has proved doubly treacherous to women.

5. That the further increase of the power of the profession holds out a serious threat to the personal liberties of all the lay members of the community.

Should these conclusions seem just, it will remain for the reader henceforth to watch wakefully and resist steadfastly the ambitious advances of this formidable order, and (as reforms rarely proceed from within) to bring public feeling to bear from the outside world to recall medical men to their proper beneficent and disinterested work. There is yet reason to hope that by such means the practice of the Healing Art may become really and in truth, what it *ought* unquestionably to be, but is now only in the language of conventional adulation—a " Noble Profession."

[To the first issue of this paper the following remarks were appended by the Editor of the *Modern Review*]

It is not without a grave sense of responsibility that we publish the above article from the pen of an esteemed con-

tributor, who prefers to withhold his signature. Our
contributor has laid a heavy indictment against a profession
that has ever been jealous of its honourable name. Yet our
duty has seemed to us very plain. Without committing
ourselves to every view or statement to be found in
this elaborate criticism, we hold with our contributor
that public opinion has been too timid in its attitude
towards the great Profession of medicine, and that it
is of vital moment that it should become both informed
and pronounced. Hitherto a silent convention has pro-
tected the Physician and the Surgeon from the wholesome
play of criticism. Language which has been common with
regard to lawyers, and still more common with regard to
clergymen, has been held a mark of ill-breeding if applied
to doctors. It has been essential on the platform and in
the magazines to allude to the latter as this noble or honourable profession, while their legal and clerical compeers have
been subject to every kind of derogatory reference. Now
few will deny that criticism has done the clergy a world of
good. Why should it do their medical brethren any harm?

All sweeping charges against a community, however care-
fully guarded, must appear unjust. Nothing could seem
more unfair than the assaults of Jesus on the Pharisees of
his time. Many of them were upright and pious men. But
the better individuals had not stood out against the worse
or made protest against their self-seeking and hypocrisy.
So came the condemnation which the Galilean pronounced to
be divinely just. It is so in other cases. There are the best
of men among the physicians and surgeons of England. But
all are held together with tremendous force, by what some
will call a fine *esprit de corps*, and others a pernicious spirit of
trades-unionism. Hence they must be criticised as a class.

The parallel between the physician and the priest is close.
In spite of the temporary revival of a sacerdotal party in the
Church of England, the people of this country, broadly

speaking, have made up their minds that the influence of
the priest in the home is inimical to morality; and the
pretensions of the spiritual adviser to enjoy the exclusive
confidence of others men's wives and daughters can amongst
us never be very widely revived. The power of priesthood
is broken for ever. But in the doctors we have a class
of men who are more and more gaining the confidence
of the boudoir, and scrupulously honourable as multitudes
of these men are, this growing social fact is pregnant
with perils precisely parallel to those which are
generally recognised among Protestants in the hold of
priests upon the home. Nay, if there remains any truth
in the proverb, *deux médecins, un athée* (and its truth
increases rather than declines), the danger from the private
medical director exceeds that from the spiritual.

But peril from the assumption of the office of private
adviser on the part of the physician demands consideration
most of all in the case of our youths. Any one who will
make a few casual inquiries will be amazed to discover the
frequency with which medical men of high repute—men
who are admitted to the friendship of good and unsuspecting
women—offer counsel to young men and even to boys
which strikes at the root of all morality, and, indeed, can
proceed from nothing else than scepticism concerning the
very possibility of morality itself.* We speak what we
know not of one, but of many, and what no medical man
will deny, though many a medical man will revolt from the
action of his fellow practitioners as vehemently as we
ourselves. What we ask of these purer spirits in the healing
fraternity is that they will speak out on this and other
matters of professional practice, and condemn their less
honourable colleagues with no faltering tongue.—ED.

* The Bishop of Bedford, speaking on this subject at a Meeting of the
Social Purity Alliance, May 3rd, 1882, said : " I know what doctors say, and I
here publicly protest against the terrible thing that is often said by doctors to
young men—that sin is good for their health. I say God forgive those who
have said it."

www.ingramcontent.com/pod-product-compliance
Lightning Source LLC
Chambersburg PA
CBHW022032190326
41519CB00010B/1689